Juicing for Inflammation

Anti – inflammatory Nature of Juicing Fruits and Vegetables

Lionel Chris

Dedication

This book is dedicated to everyone in the globe.

Table of Contents

PAGE LEFT INTENTIONALLY

Introduction

Defending the body is the healing process that takes place after there has been an armful or irritating outcome. This is what is known as inflammation. It is the process when the body immune system swings into action in helping the body protect itself to remove destructive stimuli. It can be advantageous or otherwise.

Blending in the case of more than one fruits or vegetables or squeezing out the liquid parts gives the results that would later be called juicing. It is unique in that it makes the consumption of high volume of body requirement come so handy and consumable within the shortest of time.

.

In this book, you shall be getting the inside – out of juicing and the explanations and directions on:

- ✓ The meaning of juicing.

- ✓ Different kinds of fruits.

- ✓ The different types of and the best juicer for every individual.

- ✓ Classifications of fruits.

- ✓ The meaning of inflammation.

- ✓ The types of inflammation.

…and many more.

Chapter 1

What is juicing?

Juicing involves the extraction from fruits.

It is the process where the natural liquid contents of a fruits are extracted. It involves the separation of the liquid parts of a fruit from the solid parts. The natural liquid contents include vitamins and minerals, and this can be observed on both fruits and vegetables.

The liquid so separated differs from any other liquid needed or used to combat dehydrating in that it is rich in vitamins, minerals, antioxidants, anti –inflammatory compound and phytonutrients.

The Benefits of Juicing

Despite the age long time realisation of the benefits of eating fruits and vegetables, it was not until very recently that this has become a trend especially for the purpose of health consciousness.

Juicing can bring about real great benefits with these two major instances in view.

First, it brings about the reduction in the volume of whole fruits and veggies by helping to bring them into handier containers e. g. glass cups, bottles, etc. making it a lot easier for consumption, and as much as bunches or lots you desire is consumed apparently with less efforts compared to having to eat.

Second, in some parts of the world, the peel of some fruits which are ordinarily thrown off are considered to be medicinal. Hence, they are blended along with the juice after a thorough wash for more effective results.

Juicing is confirmed to aid loss of weight, boost immune system, remove toxins, reduce the risk of cancer and aid digestion.

In contrast, there is not been any study that proves that juicing is healthier than eating the fruits or vegetables itself.

CHAPTER 2

Different juicing methods

There are four different methods of juicing namely:

A centrifugal force juicing method, masticating juicing method, twin gear juicing method, and a juice press juicing method.

Cold-pressed juicing method

This implies that the juice has been extracted from either of fruits or vegetables as the case may be using the hydraulic method of pressing. This has been argued to yield the most juice and has been the producer of the most nutritious juice.

Under this juicing method, heat or chopping is not done for the extraction on either of the fruits or vegetables, and retention of the most nutrients is guaranteed compared to any other juicing methods.

Centrifugal Force Juicing Method

This is the separation of juice from pulp leaving the juice and the pulp in a separate container. This follows some degree of heating-up. For expected result, because of the tough cell walls of the fruits and vegetables in question, as well as not to experience wastefulness, it advisable to re-juice.

Masticating Juicing Method

This is a quality that is somewhat peculiar with popular juicers like Omega, Green Star, and Champion.

This relates to chewing and grinding of substance. It involves the process of grinding the fruits and / or the vegetables for the purpose of squishing out the juice. This approach retains a little more nutrition than some other juicing methods.

Twin Gear Juicing Method

There is single gear juicer which is less expensive compared to twin gear but also of less qualities. The twin gear which is also refers to as Triturating juicer is a description of a juicer that can perform multiple functions like rub, grind and pound on fruits and / or vegetables into particles and thereafter bring out fine juice drink.

Chapter 3

Types of Juicers and Their Differences

Juicer also refers to as juice extractor is a tool used to separate juice from fruits, herbs, leafy green and other vegetables.

The process of this separation or extraction is what is known as juicing. Extraction is carried out by crushing, grinding, and / or squeezing juice out of pulp.

Types of Juicers

Reamers

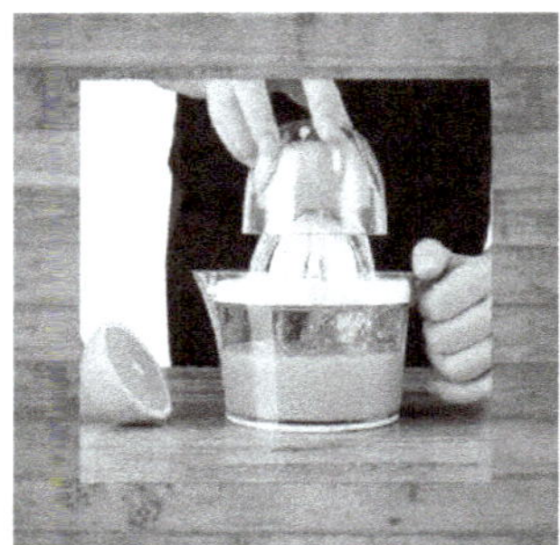

A reamer describes manual – styled squeezer used to separate citrus juice from its pulp.

Juice is extracted by cutting fruits into halves and juice is squeezed out by pressing or grinding each halves along the juicer's ridge conical centre. There are electrical reamers whose conical centre are turned automatically when fruit is positioned accordingly.

Centrifugal juicers

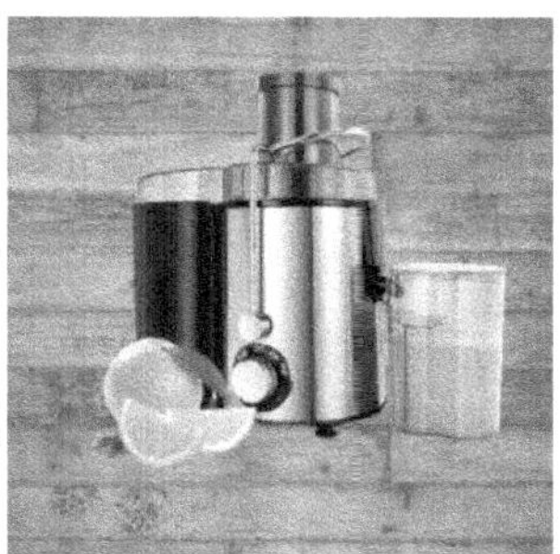

A centrifugal spins at high speed and with the flat cutting blade so designed with cuts and separates juice from pulp.

Masticating juicers

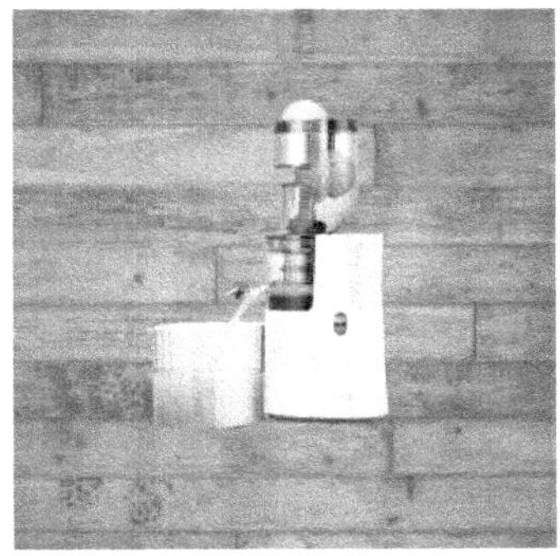

Relatively as the name implies, this juicer masticates like the teeth grind and chew. Cold press juicer or slow juicer is another name for masticating juicer. It compacts and crushes produce into smaller sections and squeezes out the juice while the pulp is thrown out via a separate outlet. Masticating juicer has more features than centrifugal.

Triturating juicers

Triturating juicer is same as twin gear juicer. This is a typical juicer that has the ability to rub, grind and pound into fine particles. Thence extract juice, nutrients, etc.

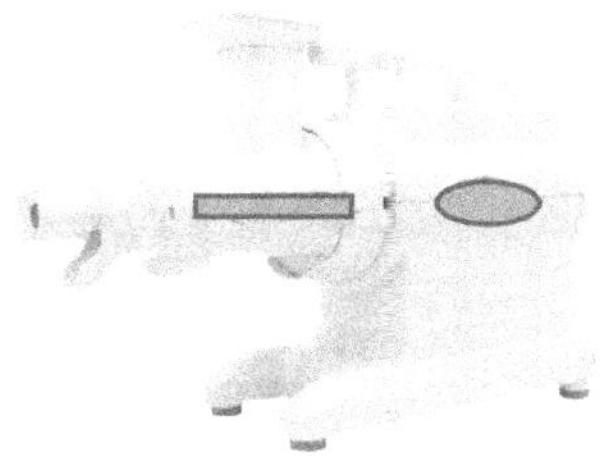

Juicing press

These are large scale press used in agricultural production. A typical juicing press can either stationary or mobile. The motive for the mobility is for usage at one orchard or the other. Juicing press is mostly used for apples

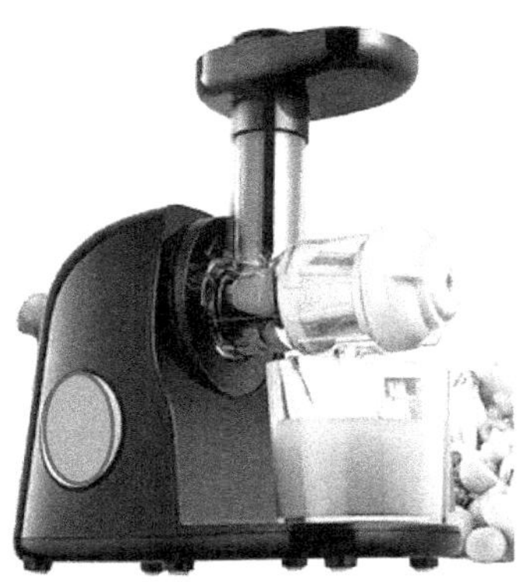

Steam juice extractor

This is a juicer that uses steaming for juice extraction. Steam juicer is a household kitchen utensil that is used to separate juice from berries, fruits and / or vegetables.

A steam juice extractor is usually a pot used to generate steam which heats its contents – berries, fruits, and / or vegetables in a punctured pot or basket that is placed on a juice collecting bowl or container on top of the steam pot.

The extraction is done without any mechanical application and the steaming makes it pasteurized therefore can be stored for longer term.

Choosing a Juicer

- What am I looking for in a Juicer

In making a choice of juicer, there are some factors to put into considerations. That is, it should be dependent on one's expectation and specification.

The consideration should include the kinds of juice one would like to make most often. There is need to consider the juicer that is best for kinds of juice you would be making. For example, when juicing for leafy juice, production of large dry pulp, and reduced produce waste, masticating juicer should be considered.

However, if your juicing would be mostly of fruits and hard vegetables, a centrifugal juicer with a high quality should be considered.

Sizes and Storage space

The size of a juicer determines the space it will be occupying which is also a function of one's kitchen and cabinet's size and easy accessibility. The horizontal masticating juicer may be able to juice out more juice but there is need to consider its weight and the possibility of moving it from the closet to the cabinet.

Whereas, the small footprint vertical juicer is best for a not too big kitchen having a limited counter space.

There also is the lightweight centrifugal model to be considered if there will always be the need to move your juicer from a point to the other (i. e. storage space to the counter).

Speed and Noise of Juicer

While you may want to consider your environment and neighbours, how fast your juicer can make juice out of your produce also needs to be considered especially if you are always on the go. You may want to consider masticating juicer here compared to centrifugal in the area of noise production but not where speed is concerned. In as quickly as 30 seconds, some centrifugal juicers can juice an apple.

Some juicers are naturally designed to be of low speed but are great when juicing soft fruits like grapes and strawberries. In like veins, high speed juicers are best for firmer produce like apples and carrots.

Ease of Use and Cleaning

Ability to operate / use a juicer easily determine how often it will be used. A juicer with easy assemblage after use for cleaning and further use will definitely get used compared to complex juicers. Truly some juicer because of their additional features of produce / items handling may require additional assemblage steps, users should still not be subjected to complex assemblage as this may lead to abandonment.

Price Value

Your investment in juicers is relatively dependent on the type of juice you desire and on how often the juicer is put to use. The prices of juicers vary between $45-$50 and $10000.

It is however advisable to consider a high quality but less expensive centrifugal juicer if you would be juicing fruits and hard vegetables.

It is worthy of notice that some juicers can work on all fruits while others may have trouble working on some fruits. This is why it is necessary to consider the juicing machine to choose.

Chapter 4

Fruits and Vegetables Juicing and Their Benefits

Benefits of juicing kale green vegetables

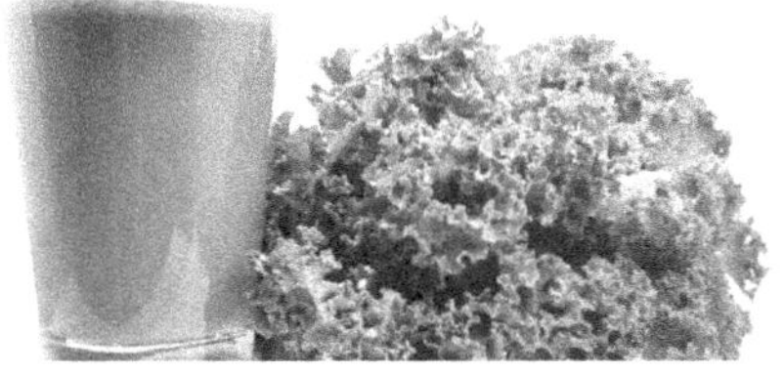

Drinking kale juice reduces risk of osteoporosis as it is associated with age. It also helps keep the bones and teeth healthy. This is because kale juice is rich in vitamin k and calcium which are needed for bone density and health.

Benefits of juicing ginger

Taking a small quantity of ginger daily can be of general good of the body system. Ginger boosts immunity and helps calm the effects of flu.

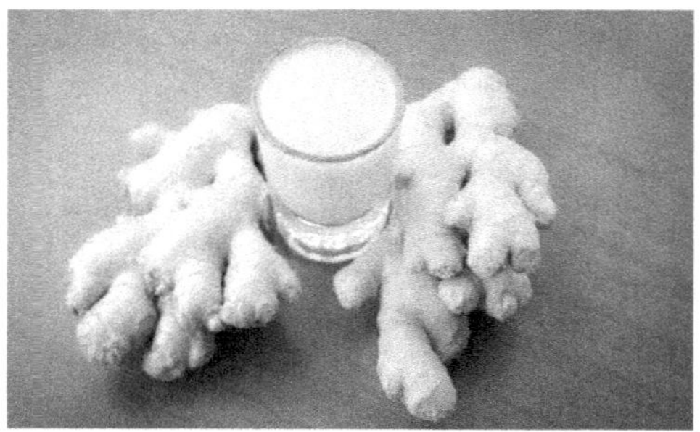

In finding solution to health issues such as indigestion, the consumption of ginger for that purpose is an excellent therapy. Ginger helps clear the digestive system as well as fights constipation.

Starting one's day with a ginger drink is a boost on metabolism.

During winter or cold season, a ginger drink helps to drive away common cold and flu because of the antibacterial properties in it. Ginger is anti-inflammatory and a great remedy for acne.

Benefits of juicing beets

Beets juicing is a product of beetroot. Beetroot can be either red or yellow.

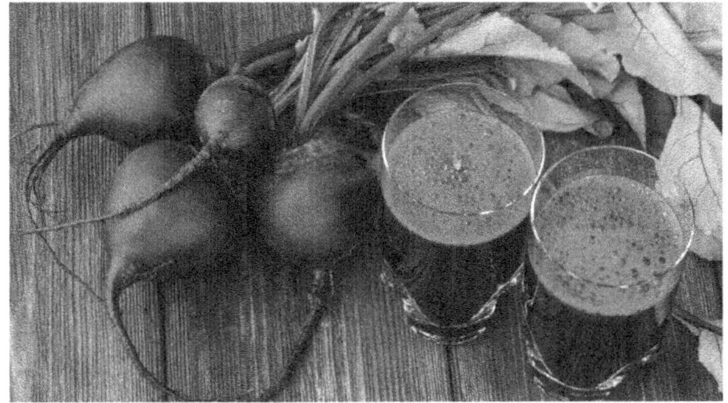

Based on research, the beet juicing has been claimed to give more energy for the day which is believed to be as a result of the presence of components to improve blood flow which has been supports for the body in responding to exercise by helping to balance the use of oxygen and an increase in gaining stamina. Beetroot juice is antioxidants.

Beet juicing can help to lower blood pressure which is guarantee through juicing because of 100% phytonutrients that will be extracted during the process of juicing.

Benefits of juicing cucumber

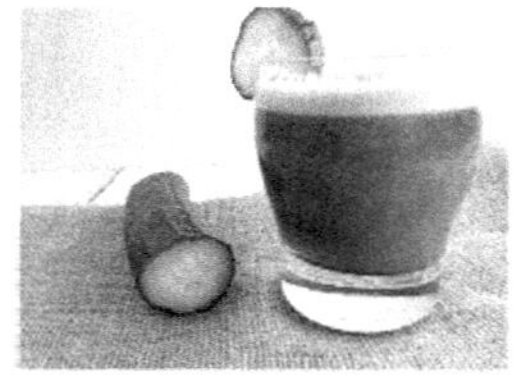

To get the best rejuvenation, you should be considering fresh cucumber juice. This is not unconnected to cucumber juice richness in nutrients such as vitamins, C, K, magnesium, silicon, potassium, etc. and for being highly a hydrating and alkalizing drink. Because of its ability to transport nutrients and hydration deep into the body cells and tissues, and the presence of electrolytes, it is a superb way to hydrated the and detoxifies the entire body system.

Cucumber juicing aids the excretion of wastes passing through the kidney as well as helps to dissolve accumulated acidic contents such as bladder and kidney stones.

Chapter 5

Making Your Own Juice

It can be both fun and simple to make fresh fruits and vegetable juice at home. This can be achieved using either juicer or blender – smoothies. Whether as juicing or smoothies, both have highly nutrients concentration and help to detoxify body system.

Making juice without a juicer is quite possible and the same rules apply in having a balanced juice.

Fruits and Vegetables for Juicing

Fruits and vegetables are categorised into soft and hard in the world of juicing. Below are the categories

Soft Fruits

PINEAPPLE
MANGO
MELONS
CITRUS
BERRIES
GRAPES
TOMATOES
KIWIS
PEACHES
PLUMS

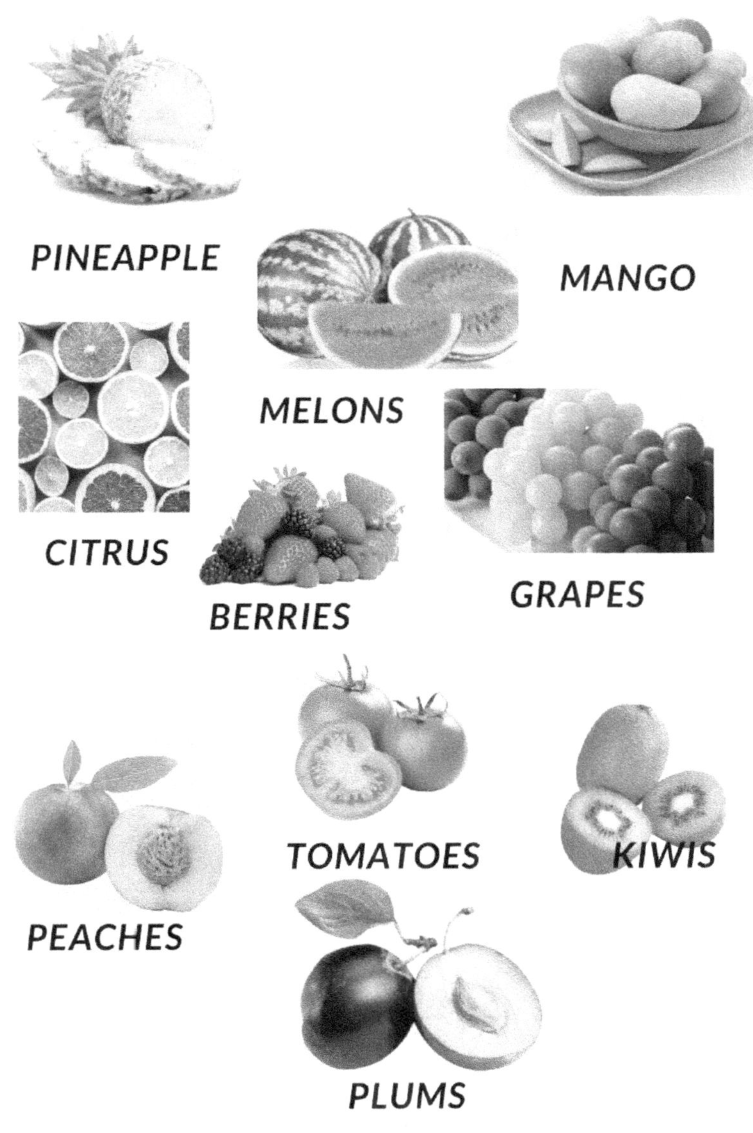

Hard fruits

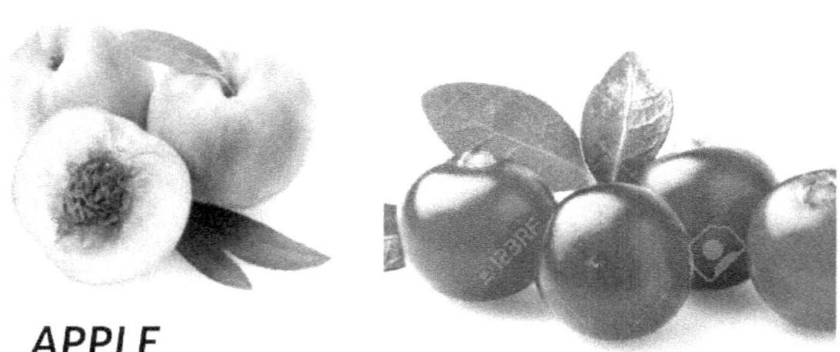

APPLE

CRANBERRIES

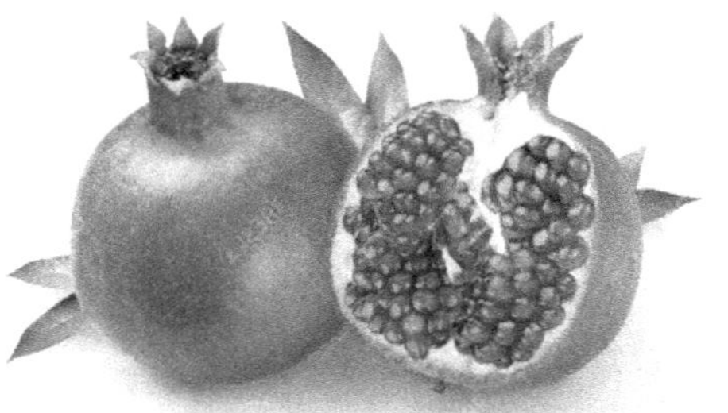

POMEGRANATE

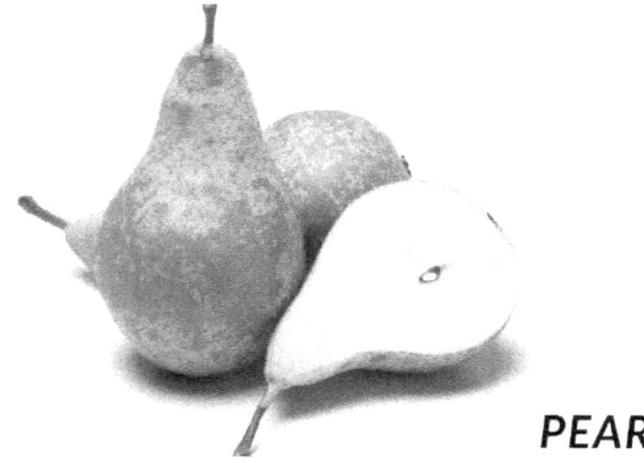

PEARS

Soft Vegetables

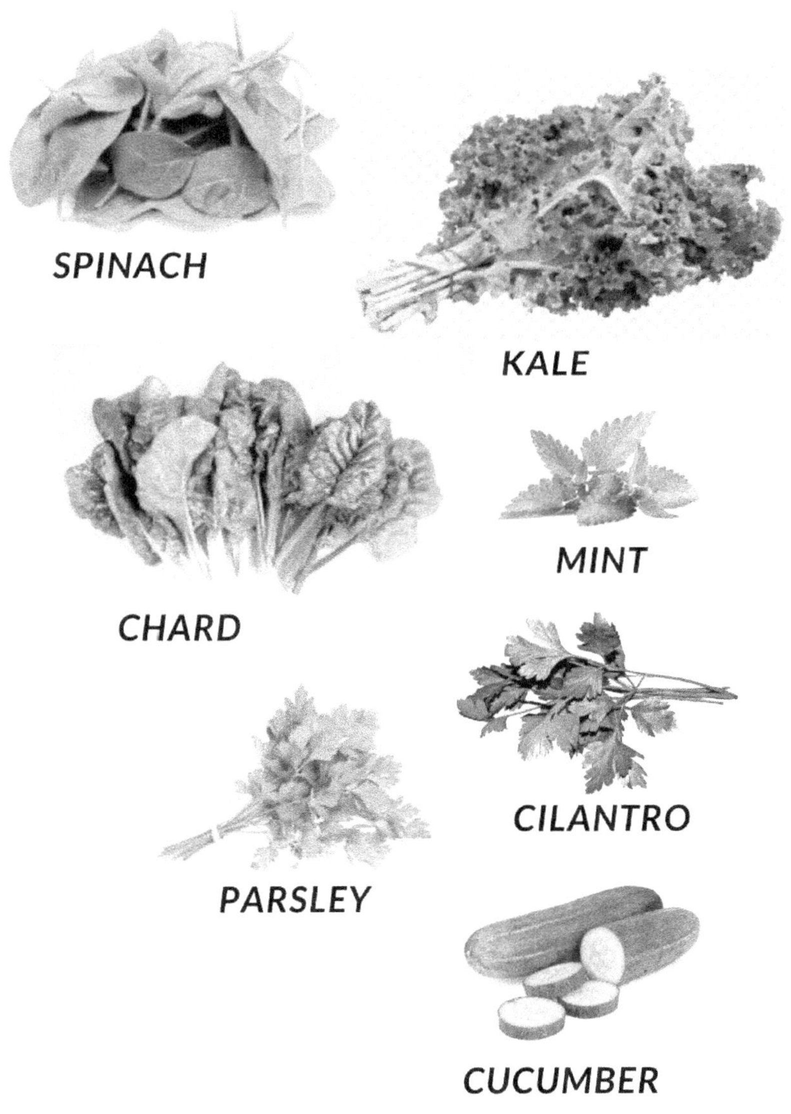

Hard Vegetables

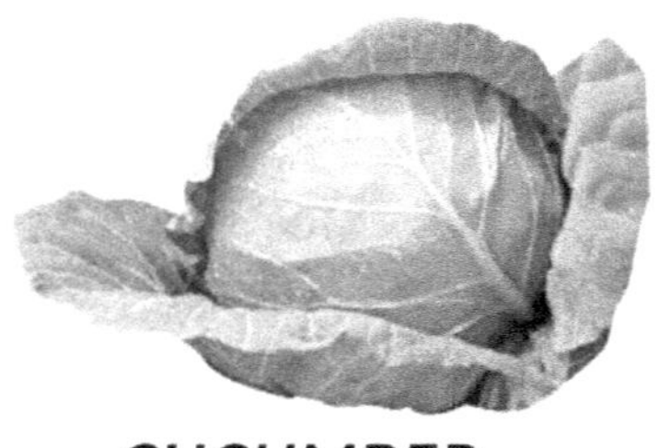

CUCUMBER

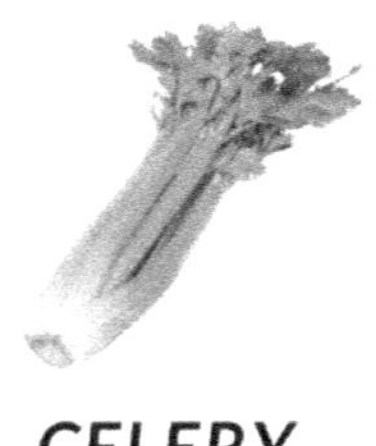

CELERY

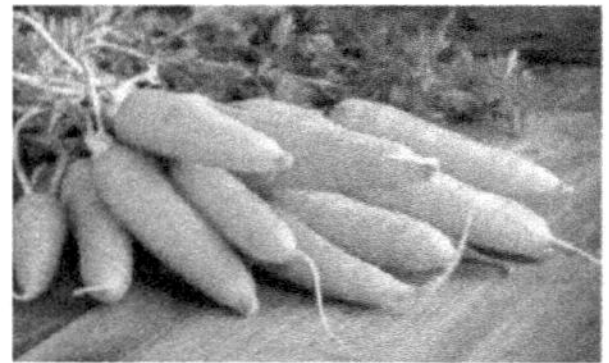

CARROTS

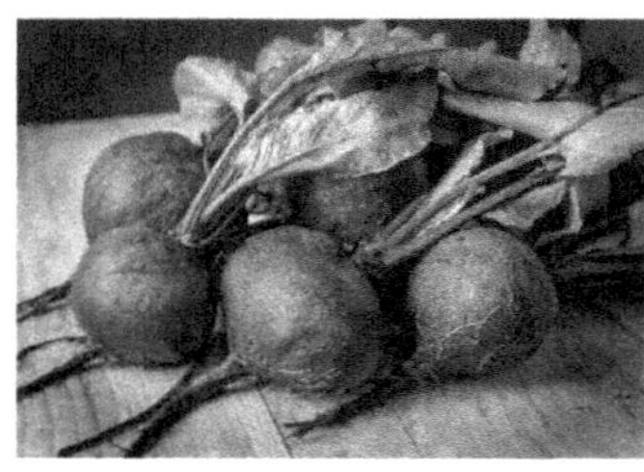

BEETS

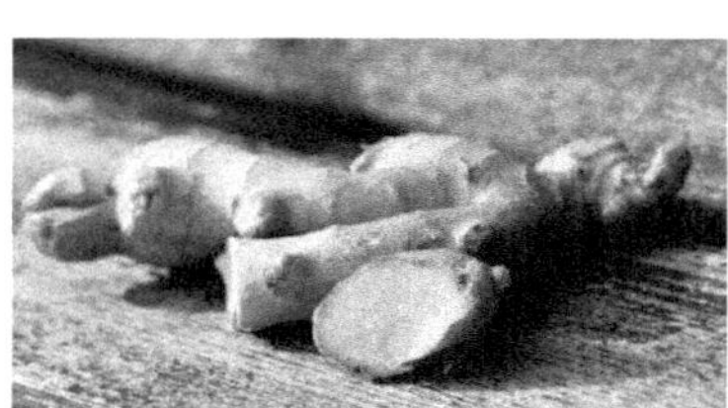

GINGER ROOT

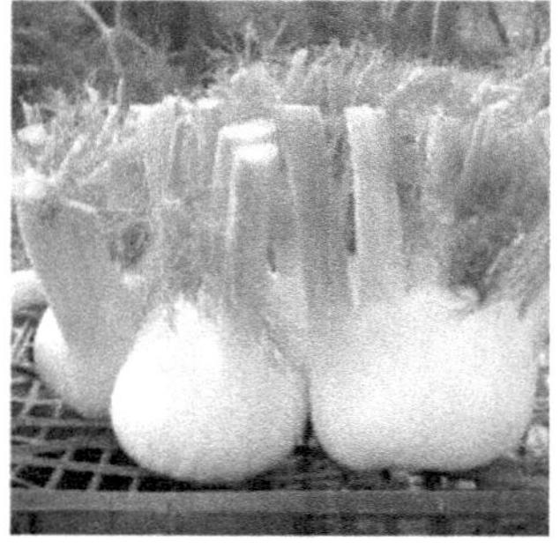

FENNEL

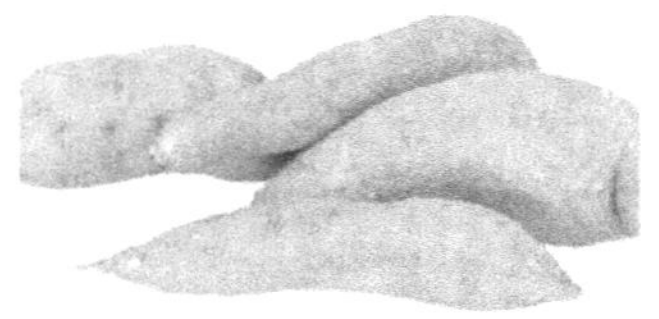

SWEET POTATO

Unfriendly juicing fruits & vegetables

The do not bring out enough liquid.

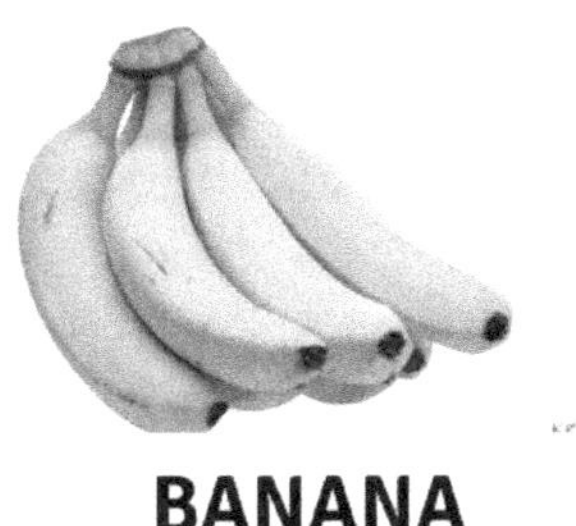

BANANA

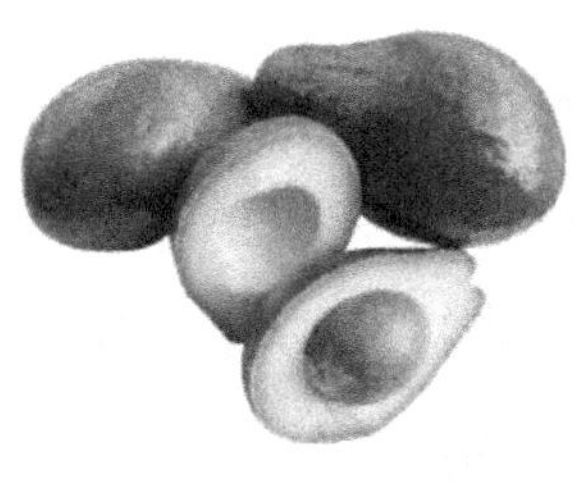

AVOCADO

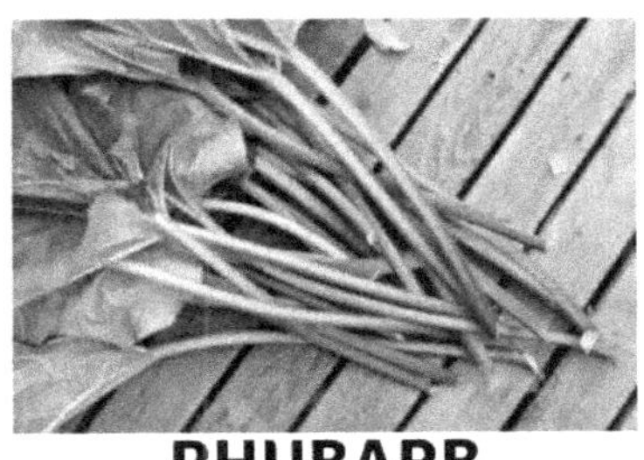

RHUBARB

Chapter 6

What is inflammation?

Inflammation can be described as one of the complex biological reaction of the body tissue to harmful stimuli such as pathogens, damaged cells, or irritants. It is also a protective reaction that comprises immune cells, blood vessels, and molecular mediators. Among other functions, inflammation as eliminator of primary source of injury to the cells, it clears out some cells and tissues that have been damaged from the original injury and inflammatory procedure. Also, it establishes tissues repairs.

Summarily, inflammation serves as the defence and repair mechanism in the body recognising and initiating healing process of damaged cells, irritants and pathogens.

This is usually accompanied by some uncomfortable signs and symptoms but this is an indication that the body is making efforts at self-healing. Without inflammatory responses, damaged cells and tissues and infections would not be able to heal.

If inflammation is of the acute class, five signs would be noticed which are heat, pain, redness, swelling and immobility which only apply to inflammation of the skin. Where inflammation happens somewhere in the internal organs, just some of these signs would manifest. This is not unconnected to the fact that some infected internal organs may not have sensory organs ending where there could be pain e.g a certain types of lung inflammation.

In contrast, chronic (or prolonged) inflammation is a long term inflammation, where during the process of inflammatory process, is characterized by instantaneous damage and healing of the tissues. This can last for several months or years and leads to gradual shift of cells especially from the site of inflammation. Chronic inflammation is linked to hay fever, periodontitis, atherosclerosis, cancer, rheumatoid arthritis, and some other several diseases despite the fact that inflammation is needed for damaged tissues to heal. It can be as a result of inability to remove the cause of inflammation, mistaken auto-immune disorder that attacks normal healthy tissues for diseases causing pathogens; a long time exposure to low level of particular irritant such as industrial chemical.

Here are examples of diseases that consist of chronic inflammatory conditions: active hepatitis, asthma, chronic peptic ulcer, periodontitis, rheumatoid arthritis, sinusitis, tuberculosis, etc.

Kindly be informed that inflammation is not same as infection. Rather, it is a part of healing process. It describes the body's reaction and response to pains and injuries. Hence, inflammation forms the process of healing.

Below is a tabular description of the differences between an acute inflammation and a chronic inflammation.

	ACUTE	CHRONIC
AGENTS OF CAUSES	Dangerous bacteria/tissue injury	Pathogens that cannot be broken down, virus infection, foreign bodies retained in the system, autoimmune responses
MAJOR CELLS INVOLVED	Primarily: neutrophils Inflammatorily: basophils and eosinophils Response from helminth worms & parasites: mononuclear cells	Monocytes, macrophages, lymphocytes, i.e mononuclear cells & fibroblasts.
ONSET	Fast	Slow
DURATION	A few days	Months to years
OUTCOMES	Inflammation improves, turns into an abscess, or becomes chronic	Tissues destroyed, fibrosis, necrosis

The Symptoms of Inflammation

The symptoms of inflammation is dependent of acute or chronic reaction. Where the reaction of an acute inflammation may include pain, redness, immobility, swelling, etc. the symptoms for chronic inflammation may include abdominal pain, chest pain, fatigue, fever, joint pain, mouth sores, rash, etc.

Causes of Inflammation

The immune system is designed to respond to physical injury and / or infection, these physical reactions leads to inflammation. This does not necessarily imply that there is an infection, nevertheless, inflammation can be caused by infection.

There are three processes that bring about noticing or suspecting inflammation. These processes may occur before or during inflammation – acute and are described below:

When supplying blood to the injured area, the small divisions of arteries become enlarge and results in blood flow increasing.

Capillaries find it easier for liquids, solutions / and or juice and proteins to move between blood and cells

A type of white blood cell called neutrophils which is filled with tiny sacs that contain enzymes and digest micro-organisms are released.

Chapter 7

Managing Inflammation

Inflammation needs to be well managed as much as it often hurts and causes stiffness and restricted mobility. People with inflammation feel different pains ranging from stiffness, discomfort, distress, agony. These pains can be any of throbbing, pulsating, stabbing or pinching. Whichever one it is, it is constant and steady.

The pain experienced as a result of inflammation is primarily because the swelling drives in contradiction to the sensitive nerve endings. The brain therefore gets pain signals.

Fruits and Vegetables for The Treatment of Inflammation

Juicing out from fruits and vegetables has proven to be a great remedy to inflammation as anti-inflammatory hormones are triggered and the release of antioxidants properties. These are needed in preventing the gathering of free radical. Vitamins and phytochemicals which are needed essentially in preventing inflammation are found in loads in a well prepared juice.

Bromelain aids digestion and helps fight back health issues like allergies, asthma and joint pains. Bromelain is found pineapple and very good at reducing pain and inflammation.

Known as nutritious leafy vegetable, kale has been mentioned to be a great source of folate, iron, magnesium, protein, phosphorus, riboflavin and vitamins (A, C, K & B6) needed for anti-inflammatory effects.

Apples have on their skin great antioxidant ingredients that can naturally act as anti-inflammatory.

Perhaps the greatest when it comes to anti-oxidants, blueberries are tested and ranked as the best solution for antioxidant activities. The blueberries have been known to be high in anthocyanin which helps to reduce inflammation.

Comprising of more than 90% liquid and full of calories, drinking watermelon juice is a guarantee of good intake. Water melon is high in antioxidants most important of which is vitamin C which helps prevents cell damage from free radicals. There are other classes of plant compounds like carotenoids and cucurbitacin E with antioxidants and anti-inflammatory effects.

Ginger, basil, tomatoes, oranges and leafy vegetables and other all help prime the immune system and reduce the risk of inflammation.

Ginger has been in used for over 4000 years ago in treating several health issues. It is most effective acting as anti-inflammatory agent helping to reduce joints inflammations. According to studies, because of its antioxidants properties, ginger juice exposes one to less pain and other inflammatory diseases as well as increase in the flow of fresh blood by getting rid of damaging impurities in the body. For more about ginger see previous chapter.

Chapter 8

Mistakes to Avoid in Juicing

It is necessary for the body to enjoy varieties of enzymes and nutrients. Therefore, make sure not to be fixed on a particular juice blend; make different kinds of juice.

In avoiding exposing oneself to another ailment while attending to one, it is advisable to stay away from piling up different fruits as this may result consuming too much sugar.

Every consumable needs to be well cleaned before taken to prevent the error of consuming pesticides. It is therefore considered a great mistake not to wash or clean your fruits before juicing them for consuming.

When some juices are not taken as when due after blending, they change concentration (they become fermented). Coupled with the fact that fresh juice is best consumed as soon as they are ready for consumption, it is a mistake to delay drinking up a fresh juice as at when ready.

The regular and real meal should not be replaced with juice.

Intake to the body has its limit. Always let your body dictate the quantity while you ensure the quality of the fruits and vegetables juice you take in. you should also take cognisance of the best time to take juice. It will be a mistake not to listen to your body.

About The Author

Lionel Chris is a dedicated and passionate author. Writes on all areas of life – government, health, fitness, economics, business, fiction, poetry and others. Always craving to improve the world through writing and various other natural arts.

Acknowledgement

I have always wanted a platform where I would be able to express some views and share knowledge and experiences. I had imagined different windows to do this without knowing how, where and when to start until I met *Brownie!* Beside putting it down, she is everything about me writing and publishing.

I am eternally grateful to *Kay* for accommodating me to every end that I enjoy.

To everyone at *Apartment I, BA*. Al they see in me is a family and relative.

Finally, to TMI, TT, TS and TM. Love you guys.